Cancer Demystified

By

David O'Halloran

Contents

Table of Contents

Acknowledgements

I understand that no small group of people can have expertise in all branches of oncology. While attempting to bring together my combined years of experience in clinical, academic and private settings, I have been privileged to meet many people – not least of all clinical coders, multi-disciplinary team coordinators, clinical audit staff, medical secretaries, researchers, cancer managers, charity-based staff, clinical trials personnel and others (you know who you are!). These people have taught me a great deal and have helped me put this manuscript together... thank you.

A huge thank you, also, to Philip Wilson from MedArt (www.medart.co.uk), who did a brilliant job with the illustrations for this book, and to freelance editor Becky Norman, who gave feedback on, reworded and amended the text in such a positive way.

Preface

Oncology, the study of cancer, is a field that is one of the most rapidly developing of all medical specialities. It is also a subject that is at the forefront of everyone's thinking, be that a cancer patient, cancer professional or government minister, and is often found at the top of governmental 'to do' lists. Many areas of the world endeavour to collect detailed and accurate information on the incidence and distribution of cancer cases, as well as information on treatment efficacy and mortality rates.

Often, those within cancer services are employed not because of their knowledge of cancer but because of other important expertise, such as administration, journalism or statistics. Those relied upon to collect cancer data, for example, tend to have little educational or clinical background on the topic. However, the changing roles and responsibilities of personnel working in this area mean that they will soon be required to have detailed knowledge of this disease. Our colleagues expect it and our cancer patients deserve it.

Cancer Demystified is born out of many years' experience educating people who deal with cancer, cancer data and cancer information in all its guises. This book speaks the language of clinicians in a way that non-clinicians can understand, providing a valuable reference to all those who work within cancer services. Currently, many oncology books on the market cover the topic extremely well but tend to be detailed and complex; indeed, without an extensive knowledge of the subject the reader can quickly become lost. Therefore, having successfully delivered education and training to those working within cancer services and charities, pharmaceutical companies, private research companies and others, I felt it was time to provide this comprehensive learning experience in text format. *Cancer Demystified* is not intended to make you a cancer expert, rather it covers the science of the disease in a way that is easily accessible. Years of teaching those from a non-cancer, nonacademic or non-science background has allowed me to tailor my teaching, bringing across important information in an understandable way. This book will be essential reading for those struggling to get to grips with cancer and its terminology, and can be used as a handy tool for comprehending and contextualising the information that you read daily. It will also provide examples of how to communicate complex information to your peers and patients alike, in a way that they can understand.

This book has been written for those who need to get 'up to speed' quickly with cancer terminology and understanding, whatever their job role. Whether you're a medical liaison officer for a pharmaceutical company who has moved into the cancer field, a journalist who has taken a new role in a cancer charity, or a multi-disciplinary team coordinator new to the field, this book is for you.

Cancer Demystified will also be of interest to those studying cancer as part of their education and training, such as student therapeutic radiographers, oncology nurses and medical students. If specialists in the field of cancer find the information in this book useful, then I am honoured. However, this book is not primarily aimed at such professionals as there are many other, more specialised works on the market that will suit their needs.

In short, this text attempts to give the reader a chance to simply and easily digest the information required for the study of cancer in a clear and concise way.

Chapter 1: Cells, tissues & cancer

With over 200 different types of cancer in existence, finding one simple definition for this disease is understandably difficult. There are, however, some important similarities among all cancers that together begin to build a picture of what the disease is. In 2000, Hanahan and Weinberg published their seminal paper 'The Hallmarks of Cancer' in the *Cell* journal. Here, they outlined six traits that appear to be common among all tumours:

1.   Cancer cells stimulate their own growth

2.   They resist inhibitory signals that might otherwise stop their growth

3.   They resist their programmed cell death

4.   They can multiply indefinitely

5.   They stimulate the growth of blood vessels to supply nutrients to tumours

6.   They invade local tissue and spread to distant sites

In 2011, they proposed two further characteristics:

7.   Cancer cells have abnormal metabolic pathways

8.   They evade the immune system

These characteristics are generally regarded as present only in abnormal cells. To understand these features of abnormal cells, and to subsequently understand how cancer forms and develops, it is necessary to take a look at what makes up a normal cell within the human body.

The cell

The cell is the basic unit of life, a building block of the human body. Each cell is surrounded by a membrane that separates it from other cells and the external environment (see figure 1). Known as the plasma membrane (or cell membrane), it acts as the cell's contact with the outside world and allows messages from this external environment to enter the cell. On the surface of the cell there are many receptors, such as the epidermal growth factor receptor (EGFR) waiting to receive these messages. These are transported by a ligand, or messenger, such as an epidermal growth factor (EGF). The ligand binds to the receptor and delivers the message, which is then transported to the nucleus of the cell via a series of specialised proteins called proto-oncogenes (e.g. Ras and Raf). Such transmission of the message is referred to as signal transduction. The message is interpreted by the DNA and the cell responds appropriately. The message might communicate to the cell to continue with its function, to stop doing its function or, indeed, to die (apoptosis). It might also communicate to the cell the need to divide (mitosis) and produce another cell. Table 1 gives some examples of ligands and receptors that are important for cell survival.

The relationship between the ligand and the receptor, and the process by which the message is brought to the nucleus, is an important process that is disrupted when a type of cancer develops. An understanding of these signalling pathways is crucial to comprehending the hallmarks of cancer as outlined above, as well as for grasping how some of the more modern treatments (e.g. targeted therapies) work. More will be said about these signalling pathways later.

The nucleus

Central to the control and functioning of the cell is the nucleus, which is responsible for cell growth, metabolism and reproduction. The nucleus is usually a round or oval organelle bounded by a membrane called the nuclear membrane. It is the largest structure in the cell. Changes to the shape and size of the nucleus are known as nuclear pleomorphism and may indicate that the cell is undergoing neoplastic change. Within the nucleus is a nucleolus containing chromosomes, of which there are 46 in a (diploid) human cell (see table 2 for an outline of the essential components of the cell).While chromosomes are complex, they are basically composed of proteins and DNA, the latter of which carries genetic information and the blue print for protein synthesis. Genes determine the characteristics of the cell and are the building blocks that make up the chromosomal DNA chains, arranged in a specific sequence on the chromosomes. Chromosomes also control cell structure, direct many of the cells' activities and contain all the genetic material essential for life. For example in some specialised cells (nerve cells), the loss of the centrosome, which contains centrioles and is found in the nucleus (see section on mitosis), means the cell cannot divide.

This is why nerve cells cannot be replaced if destroyed. Furthermore, since the cells cannot divide, they do not tend to develop into malignant neoplasms. To understand how cancer develops, it is important to consider how these genes affect the life cycle of the cell.

Figure 1: Diagram of cell

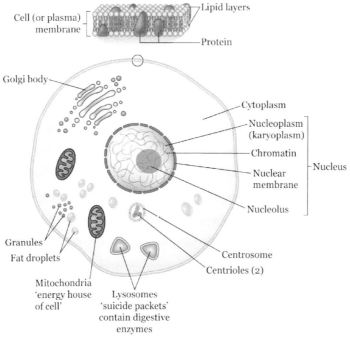

Table 1: Ligands and receptors associated with cancer

Receptor	Ligand (growth factor)	Associated cancer
Epidermal growth factor receptor: EGFR (also called HER1 or ErbB1)	EGF, transforming growth factor alpha (TGF-α), amphiregulin	Breast, bowel, lung, brain, prostate, ovarian, stomach, pancreatic, head and neck squamous-cell carcinoma (HNSCC), anal
Human epidermal growth factor receptor 2: HER2 (also called neu, EGFR2, ErbB2)	No known ligand	Breast (also some ovarian, stomach, uterine)
Vascular endothelial growth factor receptor: VEGF-R	VEGF-A, -B, -C, -D	Any cancer with a blood supply. VEGF-R is on endothelial cells lining blood vessels
Platelet-derived growth factor receptor: PDGF-R	PDGF-A, -B, -C, -D	Gliomas, gastrointestinal stromal tumours (GISTs), bone metastasis from prostate cancer; also implicated in angiogenesis
Fibroblast growth factor receptor: FGF-R 1,2,3,4	FGF	Bladder, cervical, multiple myeloma, prostate, small cell lung cancer, breast cancer, stomach cancer; also important in angiogenesis

Table 1: Ligands and receptors associated with cancer (cont.)

Receptor	Ligand (growth factor)	Associated cancer
Insulin-like growth factor-1 receptor: IGF1-R	IGF-1,2	Bowel, prostate, breast, lung; strongly inhibits apoptosis; associated with resistance to EGF-R inhibitors and chemoresistance
(c-)KIT	Stem cell factor (SCF)	GIST, small cell lung cancer, acute myeloid leukaemia, T cell lymphoma, testicular germ cell, melanoma
Fms-like tyrosine kinase 3: FLT3	FLT3 ligand	Acute myeloid leukaemia

Table 2: A summary of the most important cell constituents (not comprehensive)

Name of organelle	Function	Oncological implications
Nucleus	Controls centre of cell responsible for replication	Source of genetic material; if wrong instructions are given mutations can occur, possibly leading to tumour development
Plasma membrane / cell membrane	Allows substances of certain sizes to travel into and out of the cell; limits size and gives structure to cell; if membrane is ruptured then cell life is not viable	Cells lose their normal cell inhibition; leads to a build-up of cells (proliferation); may lead to tumour growth
Protoplasm (known as cytoplasm in cell; known as nucleoplasm in nucleus)	Contains ions, amino acids, proteins, water	Change in normal ratio of nucleus size to amount of cytoplasm can indicate carcinogenic changes; normal mature cells have low nucleocytoplasmic ratio (N:C), many tumour cells have a high N:C ratio
Nucleolus	Synthesises proteins	Inappropriate proteins may be produced

Table 2: A summary of the most important cell constituents (not comprehensive) cont.

Centrosome	Essential for early stages of cell division; forms structure to support division	Mutations in the cell may disrupt normal cell division
Chromatin masses / threads	As thickened threads, chromosomes composed of helical double chains of DNA carry genes that are essential for heredity	Any interference in the synthesis of DNA can cause the development of tumours; radiotherapy and chemotherapy can be effective as the cell is sensitive at this phase
Vacuoles	Transport waste substances out of cell or cell-produced secretions	If cell is undergoing carcinogenic changes

The cell cycle

Most of the organelles mentioned in table 2 maintain the function of the cell on a day-to-day basis. However, during a human lifetime, millions of cells are produced and millions are lost as cells are damaged, destroyed or die.

New cells are constantly needed to replace those that have been lost. It is estimated that in two hours 4 million red blood cells die and 4 million grow to replace the lost cells. To maintain the normal balance of cell numbers, cells must go through a cycle (see figure 2) that consists of duplicating all organelles and chromosomes and results in the division of two identical daughter cells.

Cells with a nucleus are referred to as eukaryotes. A eukaryotic cell cycle can be divided into two stages: interphase and mitotic (M) phase. During interphase the cell grows, accumulating nutrients needed for mitosis (cell division). This is where duplication of DNA occurs. During the M phase the cell splits itself into two daughter cells; these will then enter interphase to begin the process again.

Interphase allows the cell time to gather the nutrients it needs to enter mitosis and produce another cell. It is a phase of preparation, in which a series of changes takes place making the cell capable of division once again. Typically, interphase lasts for at least 90% of the total time required for the cell cycle, and can be divided into three consecutive phases: G, S and G2 (see table 3).

Normal cell division

Mitosis is a process whereby a single parent cell duplicates itself. It ensures that the two daughter cells are produced with the same number of identical chromosomes as the parent cell. After this process, the two daughter cells possess the same hereditary material and genetic potential as the parent cell. This kind of cell division results in an increased number of cells, so that dead and injured cells can be replaced and new cells added for body growth.

Figure 2: Diagram of cell cycle and cell phases

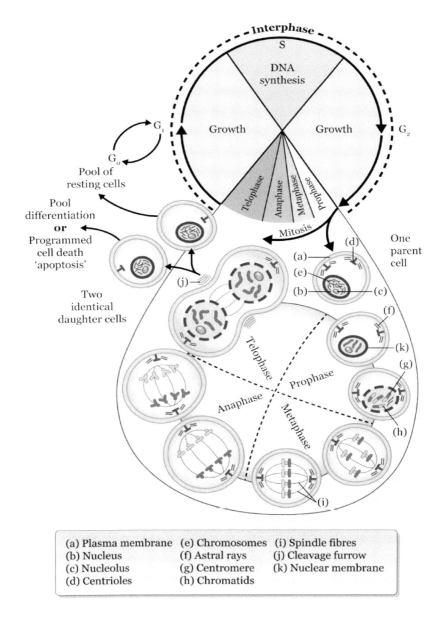

(a) Plasma membrane	(e) Chromosomes	(i) Spindle fibres
(b) Nucleus	(f) Astral rays	(j) Cleavage furrow
(c) Nucleolus	(g) Centromere	(k) Nuclear membrane
(d) Centrioles	(h) Chromatids	

Table 3: Phases of the cell cycle

Phase		Description
Resting	Gap 0 (G0)	Cell carrying on with the normal functions. It may remain in this phase for long periods of time, possibly indefinitely, as is often the case for neurons, and cells that are fully differentiated. Some cells, (hepatocytes (liver cells)), enter the G0 phase semi-permanently. Others do not enter at all and continue to divide, such as epithelial cells.
Interphase	Gap 1 (G1)	The 'initial growth phase'. Internal activities of the cell increase in rate. The cell increases its supply and production of proteins and cellular organelles, enabling it to grow. The G1 checkpoint control mechanism ensures that everything is ready for DNA synthesis.
	Synthesis (S)	The S phase is completed quickly. DNA is unwound and subsequently replicated. During DNA replication, the base pairs (cytosine, thymine, guanine and adenosine) are exposed and easily damaged by external factors
	Gap 2 (G2)	The cell continues to grow and small repairs may take place. The G2 checkpoint ensures that everything is ready to enter the M phase and divide.
Cell division	Mitosis (M)	Cell growth stops. The focus is now on orderly division into two daughter cells. A checkpoint in the middle of mitosis (the metaphase checkpoint) ensures that the cell is ready to complete cell division.

Ultimately, the cell will differentiate into the type of cell it is designed to be. Differentiation is a term that is familiar to all those working in the cancer field, where malignant neoplasms might be described as either well or poorly differentiated.

Cells produced through the process of cell division are built in a slightly immature format, and so a process of maturation (differentiation) needs to occur. When a cell has fully matured into the cell it was intended to replace it is referred to as 'well differentiated'. If it does not reach that level of maturation, then it is referred to as 'poorly differentiated'. So how does this work with tumours?

If, when analysing the cells of a malignant neoplasm down a microscope, they appear similar to normal cells, then they can be described as being well differentiated, as they have gone a long way down the process of maturation (differentiation). If, however, the cells of the malignant neoplasms look bizarre and nothing like the normal counterpart (pleomorphic), then they can be described as being 'poorly differentiated'.

To demonstrate this further we can use a sheet of paper (figure 3). The first sheet of paper (A) is a normal sheet of paper (a normal cell), ideal for printing. It looks and behaves exactly as you would expect a sheet of paper to look and behave… it is well differentiated. The second sheet of paper (B), however, is slightly crumpled (a malignant tumour cell). While it looks similar to the normal sheet of paper, the chances of causing a printer jam are significantly higher.

Although paper B is not behaving in quite the same way as paper A, it is almost behaving normally. It could be used to write a note or shopping list on, for example. This malignant cell could be referred to as well differentiated as it almost looks and behaves like the normal counterpart.

Figure 3: The sheet of paper analogy

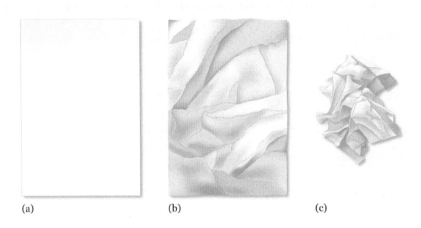

(a)   (b)   (c)

The more the paper is crumpled, the less normal it looks. As a small, scrunched up paper ball (C), it is now as far away from normal as it can be. It is no good for printing or writing on. This cell is poorly differentiated as it neither looks nor behaves like its normal counterpart.

Throwing the normal sheet of paper (the normal cell) results in it not going very far. But when throwing the crumpled piece of paper (the poorly differentiated malignant cell) it acts more like a ball and goes much further. The poorly differentiated cell does not have the characteristics of the normal cell, but has now assumed other characteristics; it behaves much better as a missile, for example. It is these new characteristics that will give this poorly differentiated cell the ability to spread (metastasise). From this analogy, it can be seen that there is a link between the level of poor differentiation and the likelihood of metastasis.

The concept of differentiation within a malignant tumour is referred to as the 'grade' of a tumour (see figure 4) and will be covered in more detail later.

Tissues

Cells of a similar type will group together to form a band of cells that are referred to as a tissue. Tissues wrap around each other to form body organs, which attach to each other to form body systems. These systems work together for the whole body. Such is the level of organisation within the human body.

Each specific tissue, along with their intercellular substance, function together to perform a specific activity, such as protection and support, producing chemicals (enzymes and hormones) or moving food through organs. Tissues can be grouped into several major categories, including epithelial, connective, muscular and nervous tissue.

Figure 4: Differentiation and the likelihood of metastasis

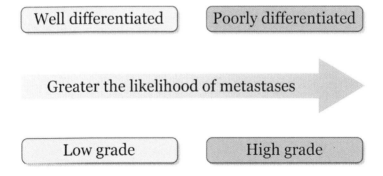

Development of tissues from cell types

There are four basic tissues of the body:

- General supporting tissues, collectively called the mesenchyme: connective tissue containing fibroblasts that form collagen fibres and associated proteins for bone, cartilage, muscle, blood vessels and lymphatic vessels

- Organ-specific cells: epithelium and specific cells for organs such as skin, intestine and liver

- Defence cells: reticuloendothelial cells are a wide group of cells derived mainly from precursor red and white cells in the bone marrow; some cells are also distributed about the body as free cells and others as fixed organs such as lymph nodes and the spleen

- Nervous system: central nervous system (brain and spinal cord) and peripheral nervous system

Epithelial tissue

Epithelial tissue covers body surfaces (such as skin), lines body cavities and forms glands (see figure 5). It forms the outer covering of the body and some internal organs. It also lines body cavities and the inner lining (mucous membrane) of the respiratory tract, gastrointestinal tract, blood vessels and ducts.

Epithelium can be arranged in single (simple) or several (stratified) layers; these cells are held together by specialised fibres and substances (for example, a basement membrane). Epithelial tissue can be sensitive to stimuli, such as taste and smell, but is avascular (has no blood supply) and receives nutrition by diffusion.

Normal features of epithelial tissue include:

- Closely packed cells

- Little or no intercellular material (matrix)

- Continuous sheets: single or multi-layered

- Nerves that may extend through the sheets, but blood vessels that do not

- Vessels supplying nutrition and remove waste (blood and lymphatics) that lie in underlying connective tissue

Epithelium overlies and closely adheres to connective tissue. The junction between the connective and epithelial tissue is a thin extracellular layer called the basement membrane from which epithelial layers develop. In malignant epithelial neoplasms, penetration (or invasion) of the tumour through the basement membrane gives the tumour the potential to spread to other parts of the body.

Figure 5: Different epithelial tissues

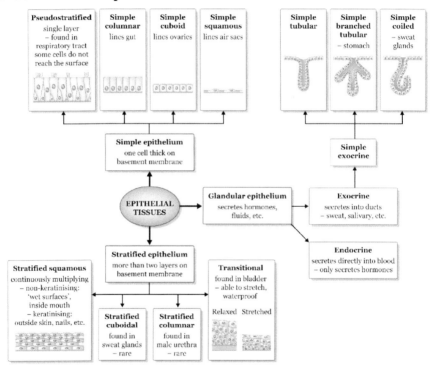

Table 4: Classification of epithelial tissue

Epithelial tissue	Cell shape	Appearance	Arrangement and function
Simple	Squamous Cuboidal Columnar	Flat, scale-like Cube like Rectangles set on end	Single layers; delicate; found in areas of absorption and filtration; occurs where there is little wear and tear
Stratified	Squamous Cuboidal Columnar Transitional	Same as above Bottom layer of cuboidal or columnar, middle layer of cuboidal and a superficial layer of cuboidal or squamous epithelium, allows expansion and can be waterproof e.g. bladder	Made of at least two layers that can withstand wear and tear
Pseudo-stratified	Squamous Cuboidal Columnar	Appears as many layered cells	Single layer but appears multi-layered; not all cells are in contact with outer surface
Glandular (secretory)	Squamous Cuboidal Columnar	Classified structurally; simple ducts or compound ducts that are branched (e.g. gastric and uterine); coiled tubular (e.g. sweat glands)	Single, or groups of, epithelial cells that function to produce secretions e.g. hormones, saliva, enzymes

Connective tissue

Connective tissue fills the spaces between organs and tissues, providing structural and metabolic support for other tissues and organs. Connective tissue is made up of cells and the extracellular matrix. The extracellular matrix is made up of fibres in a protein and polysaccharide matrix, secreted and organised by cells in the extracellular matrix. Variations in the composition of the extracellular matrix determine the properties of the connective tissue. For example, if the matrix is calcified it can form bones or teeth. Specialised forms of the extracellular matrix also make up tendons, cartilage and the cornea of the eye. General connective tissue is either loose or dense, depending on the arrangement of the fibres. The cells sit in a matrix made up of glycoproteins, fibrous proteins and glycosaminoglycan, which have been secreted by the fibroblasts. A major component of the matrix is water.

Connective tissues are defined by three main components: fibres (except for blood), ground substance and cells. All are immersed in the body's fluids and can be broadly divided into connective tissue proper, special connective tissue and a series of other, less classifiable types of connective tissues (see figure 6).

Fibroblasts are the cells responsible for the production of some connective tissues. Connective tissue is derived from mesenchyme cells that have broken away from the embryonic mesoderm. These mesenchymal cells distribute themselves widely, becoming the most abundant tissue in the body. Some mesenchymal cells remain in an undifferentiated state in the adult, but the majority differentiate into cells that share a number of characteristics. As the name suggests, connective tissue serves as a connecting system binding all other tissues together, and its functions are to bind, protect and support organs. It can be categorised both as bone tissue, which includes cartilage, and soft tissue, such as muscular, nervous, fat or fibrous tissue. Connective tissue has a rich blood supply; in other words, it is highly vascular except for cartilage, which is avascular.

Figure 6: Types of connective tissues

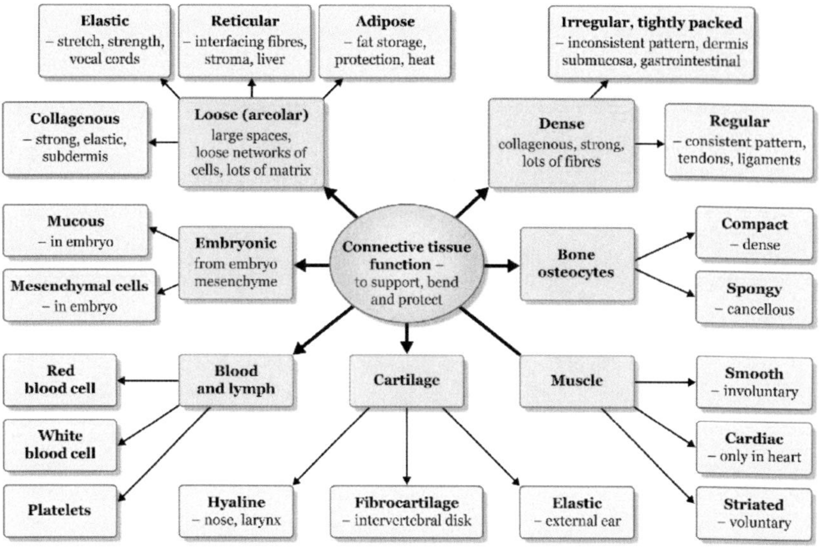

Elastic
– stretch, strength, vocal cords

Reticular
– interfacing fibres, stroma, liver

Adipose
– fat storage, protection, heat

Irregular, tightly packed
– inconsistent pattern, dermis submucosa, gastrointestinal

Collagenous
– strong, elastic, subdermis

Loose (areolar)
large spaces, loose networks of cells, lots of matrix

Dense
collagenous, strong, lots of fibres

Regular
– consistent pattern, tendons, ligaments

Mucous
– in embryo

Embryonic
from embryo mesenchyme

Connective tissue function –
to support, bend and protect

Bone
osteocytes

Compact
– dense

Mesenchymal cells
– in embryo

Spongy
– cancellous

Red blood cell

Blood and lymph

Cartilage

Muscle

Smooth
– involuntary

White blood cell

Cardiac
– only in heart

Platelets

Hyaline
– nose, larynx

Fibrocartilage
– intervertebral disk

Elastic
– external ear

Striated
– voluntary

Features of normal connective tissue:

- The cells are widely scattered within large quantities of an intercellular substance referred to as the matrix; the cells of the tissue secrete this.

- The matrix of the tissue determines the qualities of the tissue; for example, fluid, semi-fluid or mucoid.

- Cartilage is a connective tissue, but its matrix is firm and pliable. The matrix of bone is hard and non-pliable.

- The cells also store fat, ingest bacteria and cell debris, form anticoagulants and create antibodies to protect the tissue from disease.

For cancer to develop, normal cells must attain damage and begin to divide uncontrollably. The normal body should not allow abnormal or mutated cells to divide and, in different stages of the cell cycle, checks and balances are in place to prevent this from happening. If a cancer develops, however, then this failsafe mechanism is breached. How it is breached, and what damage is done to the cell, will be explained in the next chapter.

Chapter 2: Neoplasms and the hallmarks of cancer

Normal cell replication is under careful control in the body, but sometimes cells will undergo duplication outside the normal control mechanisms of the body. This can result in an excess of new tissue, called a neoplasm (neo = new; plasm = growth) or tumour. The study of tumours is called oncology (onco = mass, bulk; -ology = to study). To ensure that a cell is initiated and stimulated through the cycle, there are a number of specialised genes within the cell that will monitor this process. Aberrant, or malfunctioning, genes may lead to genetic instability, which is the trademark of cancer cells. And, in turn, this genetic instability may lead to the hallmarks of cancer referred to in chapter 1.

So how do genes become damaged? And what causes them to change? There are several possible mechanisms for this change (see figure 7).

Each time a cell divides it is required to replicate the DNA of the cell. DNA is extremely long and complex and, when cells are constantly requested to duplicate this structure, mistakes can be made.

Think about the entire works of Shakespeare. The simple, but laborious, task of continually copying these works word for word for many days is approximately the same amount of information that is replicated each time a cell divides. The process of copying all of his works will inevitably lead to mistakes – and it is the same for cells when dividing. Mistakes in the genes of the cell can lead to aberrant behaviour, which may subsequently lead to cancer formation.

Throughout a lifetime, the human body is exposed to many carcinogens (cancer-causing agents). For example, UV radiation, asbestos and chemicals (benzene). Such exposure over a long period of time can accumulate damage within the DNA and, once again, may lead to the development of cancer due to aberrant cell behaviour.

Figure 7: Damage to DNA

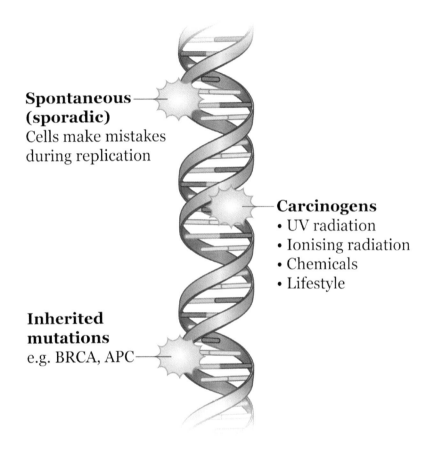

It is also known that certain damaged genes may be passed on to future generations. The *BRCA 1* and *BRCA 2* genes can be inherited by a person's mother or father. These genes produce proteins that help repair damaged DNA and therefore play a crucial role in ensuring the stability of the cell's genetic material. When either of these genes is mutated, or altered, such that its protein product is not made or does not function correctly, DNA damage may not be repaired properly. As a result, cells are more likely to develop additional genetic alterations that can lead to cancer.

Proto-oncogenes encourage and promote growth and division of cells as a response to signals from other cells (see figure 8). This involves relaying information from the cell membrane to the nucleus via the cytoplasm. If these proto-oncogenes are damaged, perhaps by a carcinogen or virus, they can mutate. This may lead to these genes being permanently switched on, which may promote over-production of growth factors and uncontrolled cell growth. The proto-oncogene is then transformed into an oncogene. Many oncogenes have been researched to date, including *ras*, *myc*, *her2* and *braf*. A knowledge of these oncogenes and their role in cancer proliferation and growth is leading to a new generation of therapy called targeted therapy, which is designed to target and stop the signal transmission.

Tumour suppressor genes, such as *TP53*, *PTEN* and retinoblastoma (*Rb*), act as guardians for the cell, monitoring for mutations. During the cell cycle, the cell is constantly checking that everything is optimal for cell division. Tumour suppressor genes are responsible for this checking process and will initiate apoptosis (programmed cell death) if there is a possibility that cell division may result in some form of mutation. If tumour suppressor genes are lost or no longer working, and therefore not monitoring for damage, the cell will be allowed to divide, even in a damaged format. Lost or inactivated tumour suppressor genes can be a common prelude to cancer or tumour development. For example, in over 50% of all tumours, the tumour suppressor gene *p53* is damaged.

Abnormal cell production may cause an accumulation of too many cells (known as hyperplasia). When this occurs, while there may be an increase in cell numbers, each individual cell appears normal (well differentiated). Hyperplasia is typical in benign neoplasms. It may also be accompanied by an increase in the size of the cells (hypertrophy), which is often a response to cell damage or destruction, or increased hormone stimulation.

Figure 8: Oncogenes, tumour suppressor genes and repair genes

- Proteins from (proto) oncogenes promote cell growth, survival and proliferation e.g. EGFR, RAS, B-Raf, HER2
- In cancer cells oncogenes are overactive, mutated or amplified thereby making too much protein

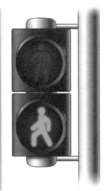
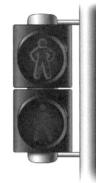

- Proteins from tumour suppressor genes stop cell growth and replication, may trigger apoptosis e.g. RB, PTEN, TP53
- In cancer cells tumour suppressor genes are lost or not working

- DNA repair genes sense damage and repair damaged DNA e.g. BRCA; sometimes classed as tumour suppressor genes
- In cancer cells DNA repair genes are lost or not working

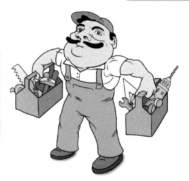

Metaplasia (meta = change; -plasia = form, growth) may occur as a result of chronic irritation. Here, the cell changes from one type of epithelium to another – one that can best deal with the irritable environment. For example, metaplasia can be seen in the lungs of smokers where the cells change from ciliated columnar epithelium to stratified squamous epithelium, which is more suited to dealing with the chronic irritation. Barret's oesophagus is a condition found in those who suffer from chronic regurgitation of stomach acid into the lower part of the oesophagus. As a result of this chronic irritation, the cells of the lower oesophagus undergo metaplastic change from squamous to columnar epithelium. Such metaplastic changes will persist if the irritation is allowed to continue and, indeed, may lead to further changes where the cells start to become even more disorganised through, for example, dysplasia and neoplasia.

Dysplasia (dys = bad, difficult) causes more disordered growth than hyperplasia. Here, the cells may demonstrate changes in cell shape, growth or differentiation (see figure 9). Dysplasia restricted to the originated tissue is referred to as *in-situ* and by definition is non- or pre-invasive.

Figure 9: Cellular changes from normal to neoplasm

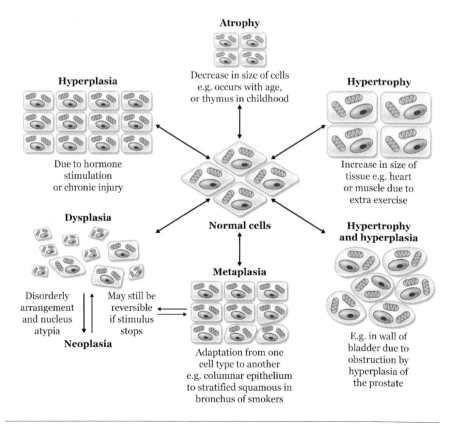

Cancer formation (carcinogenesis)

Cells of the body may accumulate random damages throughout a person's lifetime. This is why most types of cancer will occur in people over the age of 60 (see figure 10). As suggested earlier, such damage may result in an accumulation of oncogenes, promoting the growth and division of cells, as well as a loss of tumour suppressor genes, thereby allowing abnormal cells to divide and grow. Such is the 'multiple hit' process of cancer development.

In benign neoplasms, this damage and mutation is usually minor, as cells tend to only undergo hyperplastic changes. There will be more cells, but each cell appears well differentiated (normal). Because benign tumours remain localised and do not metastasise (spread), it is rare for them to cause serious health issues. An exception may be tumours in the pituitary gland. Here, the vast majority are benign, but the site of the tumour (located in the *sella turcia,* a small depression in the bony plate at the base of the skull) is potentially life threatening. As a pituitary tumour enlarges, the patient displays intracranial pressure symptoms that may have fatal implications if not treated.

Malignant neoplasms

Malignant neoplasms, on the other hand, are defined by their ability to invade local tissue and metastasise to others parts of the body. Epithelial tissue, as stated earlier, is separated from the connective tissue by a basement membrane. Epithelial tissue is avascular, meaning it does not have blood or lymphatic vessels within it. Rather, the blood and lymph vessels can be found below the basement membrane, intermingled with the connective tissue. Epithelial cells obtain oxygen and nutrients, and eliminate waste, via a process of diffusion across the basement membrane.

Figure 10: Crude rate of all cancers by age

Crude rate per 100,000, exc. NMSC*

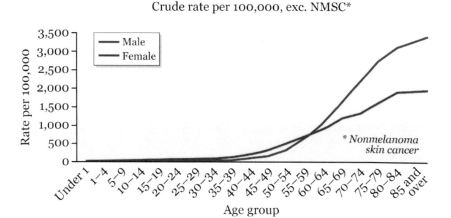

Source: Office for National Statistics 2016

As a result of damage and irritation, the epithelial cells may undergo metaplastic or dysplastic changes resulting in cells that have cancerous properties. But these cells remain confined by the basement membrane. This neoplasm is said to be *in-situ*. Referring to figure 11 only epithelial tissue has the potential for this *in-situ* phase, while, contrastingly, connective tissue is in intimate contact with blood and lymph vessels and is not separated by a basement membrane.

As the cells of the neoplasms continue to receive damage, or progressively mutate, they will begin to develop characteristics (hallmarks of cancer) that will allow them to invade through the basement membrane. When this happens, the neoplasm is said to be invasive. Such a breach of the basement membrane allows malignant cells to further infiltrate the surrounding tissue and potentially spread into the blood and lymphatic vessels.

Figure 11: Carcinoma *in situ* compared with invasive carcinoma

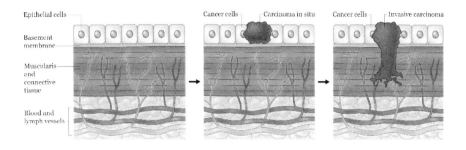

Consequently, the malignant neoplasm is able to be transported to other parts of the body, meaning it can metastasise.

A summary of the differences between benign and malignant tumours is shown in table 5.

Tumour growth

In normal cell division two daughter cells are produced. One will return to the cell cycle to be called on again (G_0), while the other will develop into a mature cell with specialised structures and functions. As mentioned in chapter 1, this process is called differentiation and is a normal procedure that the majority of cells in the body will go through. Some tissues retain the ability to divide throughout life, usually in an area prone to constant abrasion, such as the mucous membrane of the mouth. These areas require a constant supply of newly produced cells, but as cells become more specialised they may lose their ability to reproduce. Because nerve cells are highly specialised and do not replicate, tumours of true nerve cells are extremely rare. However, tumours known as gliomas do arise from glial cells, which support nerve cells.

Table 5: Differences between benign and malignant neoplasms

Benign	Malignant
Encapsulated	Not encapsulated
Grow by expansion and never invade. Produce pressure effects or systemic effects and may secrete hormones	Grow by expansion and invasion (direct spread)
Usually slow growing	Growth rate can vary
Under some normal control of body	Under no control
Remain localised	Spread from primary site (metastasise)
Cells resemble original tissue (well differentiated)	Cells have variety of presentations from well differentiated to poorly differentiated (anaplastic)
Not usually fatal, unless pressing on a vital organ	Always fatal unless treated

Tumour cells tend to divide more frequently than normal cells but, even within a single tumour, the rate of growth can vary tremendously, thus leading to different parts of the tumour demonstrating varying degrees of differentiation. When a tumour cell is well differentiated, it looks and behaves like its parent cell. The less differentiated (poorly differentiated or undifferentiated) a cell is, the more it is mutated and the less it looks and acts like the parent tissue. Assessing the level of differentiation is called grading and may be defined as an estimate of the degree of malignancy. As suggested earlier, there is a relationship between the level of poor differentiation and the greater likelihood of metastases.

Malignant tumours and the hallmarks of cancer

The ability to metastasise is the fundamental difference between benign and malignant tumours. This is what defines cancer as a disease. In the majority of cases, metastasis – rather than the primary tumour – will be the cause of death.

As malignant tumours continue to grow and divide they become increasingly mutated (poorly differentiated). As this happens they will develop certain characteristics, namely the hallmarks of cancer (outlined in chapter 1).

The more poorly differentiated a tumour cell is the more of these characteristics it will demonstrate; the more of these characteristics it demonstrates the easier it will be for it to grow uncontrollably and spread.

Cancer cells stimulate their own growth

Cells of the body are constantly receiving stimuli from other cells around them. In this microenvironment, messages (growth factors) are constantly being exchanged that promote cell growth, replication and survival.

Growth factors are responsible for initiating the signalling pathway in cells. This pathway is the cell's method by which it converts an external message to an internal response. On the surface of every cell there are receptors waiting to receive a growth factor. Each growth factor will 'fit' or bind to a specific receptor. For a list of receptors and their associated growth factors, refer to table 1 (chapter 1).

Receptors are essentially made up of two parts: an external portion, which protrudes out of the cell membrane and allows for attachment of the growth factor, and an internal portion, which protrudes inside the cell from the membrane. Such an arrangement allows for the growth factor message to be taken inside the cell. The epithelial growth factor (EGF) binds to the epithelial growth factor receptor (EGFR), as shown in figure 12. What happens next is a process called signal transduction caused by phosphorylation of downstream proteins.

Figure 12: EGFR receptor and signal transmission

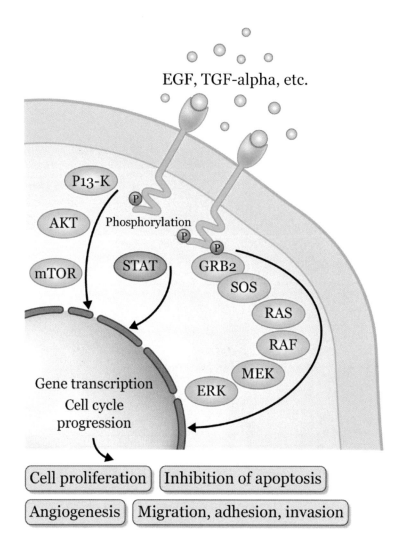

When a growth factor binds on to a receptor, it activates the internal portion. This internal portion, called the kinase, transfers a phosphate group to the next protein. Most of the proteins in these signalling pathways work by a simple on/off process. The addition or removal of the phosphate group will switch the next protein on or off. Therefore transferring the message on comprises a simple process of passing the phosphate group to the next protein, then the next, then the next, until it reaches the nucleus of the cell. Here, it can affect genes, triggering a cellular response of growth, replication and survival (see figure 13).

In a cancer cell this signalling pathway seems to be permanently switched on. How does this happen? Essentially, there are three mains ways in which a cancer cell escapes the normal signalling pathway.

Figure 13: Signal transduction

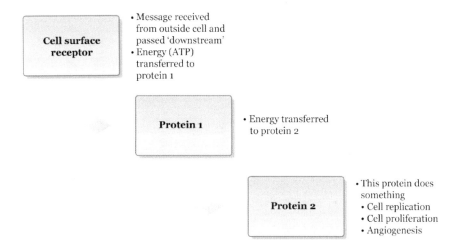

First, cancer cells are good at manufacturing their own growths factors, which leads to neighbouring cancer cells producing their own growth factors – the whole process is self-promoting. Lots of growths factors means lots of signal transduction, which means lots of cancer cell growth, replication and survival.

Second, cancer cells may modify the receptor so that it is permanently switched on regardless of whether a growth factor is present, meaning that the cancer cell's messaging system is always active. The cancer cell may also produce more than the normal number of receptors, causing hypersensitivity to any growth factors present in the tissue and resulting in more cancer cell growth, replication and survival.

Third, the proteins inside the cell that are responsible for passing on the message internally can also be permanently switched on. Such a situation means that the cell does not have to rely on the growth factor, or receptor, as the message will be started inside the cell by a faulty protein. In figure 13, above, notice the Ras protein, downstream from EGFR, inside the cell. Mutated (damaged) Ras is usually associated with aggressive diseases and poor prognosis. It is found in one quarter of all cancers and over 90% of pancreatic cancers.

Cancer, it would seem, is a consequence of this messaging system being permanently switched on. A strategy to treat cancer, then, would be to switch off this messaging system in the cancer cell. This forms the basis of targeted therapy, with the three areas mentioned above providing the targets. Inhibitors of these targets stop the message and prevent over replication and growth of cancer cells. Cetuximab is an example of such an inhibitor. Its target is the external portion of EGFR, which is overactive in many head and neck cancers, as well as colon cancer, and so the drug is routinely used in the treatment of these cancers.

Identification of suitable targets, and production of effective inhibitors, will hopefully lead to more effective treatments in the future.

Cancer cells resist inhibitory signals that might otherwise stop their growth

As previously discussed, cells must go through the cell cycle in order to replicate. Made up of phases, the cycle is the means by which a perfect replica cell is produced. In particular, DNA is replicated. Throughout this process, and before the replicating cell is able to move into the next phase, there are a series of checks and balances designed to make sure that only a perfect cell, and perfect DNA, is allowed to replicate. One very important monitor is the retinoblastoma protein (pRb).

The role of an active pRb is to bind to the E2F transcription factor and prevent the cell from advancing from the G1 phase to the S phase of the cycle. Therefore, the route to progression is simple: disassociate Rb from the E2F. The catalyst for this is a cyclin-CDK complex, which phosphorylates (addition of a phosphate groups as outlined above) Rb and makes it now inactive. Inactive Rb detaches from the E2F transcription factor, allowing E2F itself to become active and push the cell into the next phase of the cycle.

Whether or not a cell will progress through the cycle is driven by anti-growth signals. One such antigrowth signal is TGF-beta, and its presence halts the progression of the cell cycle.

It is the disruption of these pathways that allows cancer cells to continue through the cell cycle even if it is not ready to do so. Cancer cells will stop responding to the presence of TGF-beta and will stop producing receptors so that TGF-beta cannot bind on successfully. Alternatively, it will stop or ignore the downstream proteins from TGF-beta. The net result is that the cell does not receive the antigrowth signal and therefore carries on regardless.

In some cancer cells the Rb protein is lost altogether. For example, HPV produces a certain protein that binds to Rb and prevents its action. The inability of Rb to do its job, either because it is directly inhibited or because it does not receive the message, means that damaged cells – cancer cells – are able to replicate unhindered.

Loss of contact inhibition

Another anti-growth signal to consider is one that promotes contact inhibition in normal cells. When normal cells are seeded into a petri dish they begin to divide and proliferate. As the cells fill the space they start to touch one another and, consequently, begin to slow their rate of division. Such behaviour is called contact inhibition. Once the space is completely filled the rate of cell division becomes balanced with the rate of cell death, resulting in the number of cells remaining the same. Contact inhibition is the body's way of keeping cell numbers constant.

Cancer cells behave quite differently. When seeded among normal cells, all the cells will proliferate as normal until they fill up the space provided. But whereas normal cells begin to slow their rate of division as a result of contact inhibition, cancer cells do not. They continue to proliferate in an unregulated manner yielding a clump of cells referred to as a tumour (neoplasm).

Angiogenesis

As a normal part of growth, development and wound healing, the body must grow new blood vessels to oxygenate the tissues. In a process called angiogenesis, new blood vessels sprout from existing ones. On stimulation by angiogenic growth factors, endothelial cells (present on pre-existing blood vessels) break through the basement membrane confining them and begin to proliferate into the surrounding tissues, forming a sprout that will extend towards the angiogenic source. Vascular endothelial growth factor (VEGF) is an active component of this process.

Angiogenesis is also a vital process in the development of tumours. A tumour needs to grow only to a few millimetres in size before it will become oxygen deficient. As a result, it will begin to send out angiogenic growth factors such as VEGF that will diffuse through the tissue, activating endothelial cells on nearby blood vessels and leading to new blood vessel formation. An understanding of this process is leading to the development of novel targeted therapies, designed to inhibit the process of angiogenesis in tumour formation, with varying clinical results.

Loss of cellular adhesion and motility

Epithelial cells stay closely packed and joined together through a process of junctions. They are confined by their basement membrane and remain in their locale. It is now known that cancer cells undergo a transformation from epithelial cells to a more primitive mesenchymal cell (figure 14). Such a transition is called epithelial to mesenchymal transition (EMT).

Mesenchymal cells have the ability to disconnect from the surrounding cellular framework, losing their cellular adhesive qualities and becoming motile. As such, they are able to

Figure 14: Epithelial to mesenchymal transition

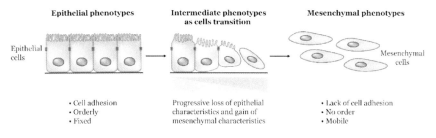

disconnect from the basement membrane and interact directly with the connective tissues around the epithelial cells. This is called invasion.

It is worth noting here that cancer cells appear to hijack what is a normal mechanism during human development within the embryo. Each human body consists of trillions and trillions of cells, and each of these cells has developed from a single blastocyte (a fusion between the ova and sperm). During the process of embryonic development, primitive cells need to be able to migrate to where they are needed and to differentiate into (become) different types of cells. This seems to be exactly what cancer cells are able to do.

Bodily tissues consist of primarily epithelial and mesenchymal cells (as discussed earlier). Epithelial cells are designed to line the insides and sometimes the outsides of body organs, offering protection (mainly) from the outside environment. Mesenchymal cells, on the other hand, are designed to move freely through the inter-cellular spaces via what is termed the extracellular matrix. Mesenchymal cells are able to differentiate into other types of cells, such as bone and cartilage cells.

Once the cancer cell has migrated to a different part of the body, it may get lodged and continue to grow and divide forming a metastasis. Interestingly, the cells of this metastasis will resemble the cells and tissues from where it has originated. For example, a metastasis in the liver that came from a primary breast carcinoma will resemble the cells of the breast rather than the liver. Hence it is further assumed that the cells of the metastasis must also undergo the reverse of EMT and transform back into the epithelial type of cell, which is referred to as mesenchymal to epithelial transition (MET).

Further research and understanding of this process will help to improve knowledge of the concept of metastasis. Drugs may be developed that can inhibit EMT and/or MET and thus prevent metastasis from occurring. If the cancer can be kept in the locale from where it originated, the primary site, treatment will be much more successful.

Methods of metastasis

The process of metastasis begins with the invasion of surrounding tissue (see table 6). Normal cells arrange themselves in tissues in neat, orderly ways with their own personal space. The growth of a normal cell continues until it touches another cell, at which point it stops. As mentioned earlier, this is called contact inhibition and is a property that tumour cells ignore. The lack of contact inhibition enables malignant cells to invade in and around other tissue, starving the normal tissue of essential nutrients and oxygen and causing normal cell death. Normal cells also demonstrate cellular adhesion, which is when cells of the same type clump together to form an organ or tissue. Malignant tumour cells lack cell adhesion, allowing them to break off from the primary tumour and invade other areas of the body. They may invade into cavities (abdominal or thoracic) or erode through blood and lymph vessels, which enables them to be carried away to distant parts of the body (see table 6). Once lodged in other parts of the body (typically brain, lung, liver and bone), the tumour cells are able to establish a new blood supply (a) and thereby continue to grow. Eventually, unless an appropriate intervention is administered, the tumour will compromise the function of the organ it is in and cause organ failure, which may lead to death.

Table 6: The spread of malignant neoplasms

Type of spread	Description of spread
Direct or local	Variable growth patterns can result in affecting organ function; lead to ulceration if on epithelial surface; produce perforation or a fistula; cause obstruction; and invade nerves, giving pain and symptoms far from the primary source.
Haematopoietic (blood) / haematogenous	Tumour cells erode through blood vessels, travel throughout the bloodstream to distant sites and form secondary tumours in organs. Common tumours that spread via blood include lung, breast, thyroid, kidney and prostate.
Lymphatic	Tumour cells erode through lymph channels, are carried along with the lymph, and lodge and grow in lymph nodes.
Transcoelomic (implantation)	Tumour cells break off from the primary and spread throughout a body cavity via the fluid in the cavity, such as in the pleural, pericardial or peritoneal cavity, and implant on any surface within.
Seeding	Tumour cells may be left in an incision after surgical intervention and allow a recurrence of the primary tumour.

The time a cell takes to go through the cell cycle and produce two identical cells is called the doubling time. For an individual tumour, the doubling time can vary enormously. As stated earlier, a neoplasm's growth is reliant on its blood supply, which initially depends on starving the adjacent tissue as the tumour grows.

Malignant tumours can secrete blood-producing factors, which can generate their own blood supply. The rate of cell death divided by the number of cells with a blood supply is known as the mitotic index.

Figure 15: Graph to illustrate growth of a tumour

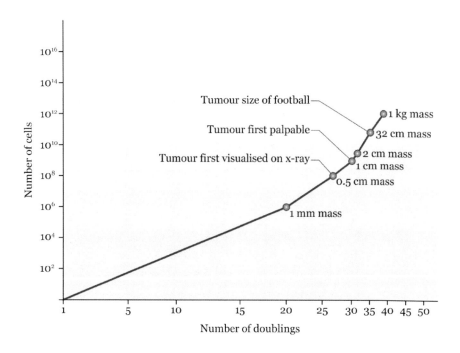

Often by the time the neoplasm can be visualised on an x-ray, which is when a mass is approximately 0.5cm in size (see figure 15 above), the monoclonal cell (meaning all cells that have been developed from one cell and are identical) will have gone through around 26 doublings. This is often the period of most rapid growth before being detectable with imaging. The tumour may only require 5 to 10 more doublings to grow from clinically palpable to systemic disease. In some cases, the neoplasm may become systemic before being clinically palpable and the patient may therefore present with metastatic disease from a primary of unknown origin.

Screening is a method whereby a malignancy can be detected before the disease becomes clinically apparent and produces symptoms. Once a tumour has been diagnosed it is important to gain as much information as possible about the particular cancer case. Such information and its uses will be covered in the following chapter.

Chapter 3: Classification of malignant tumours

Malignant tumours can be classified in a number of ways:

- Histopathological

- Locational

- Biological

- Grade and stage

Histopathological

Tumours can be classified according to their tissue of origin (see table 7).

- Tumours that develop from epithelial cells, which are found in the linings of the skin, organs, digestive tract and airways, are termed carcinomas. This is the most common cancer type, accounting for approximately 80–90% of all cancers.

- Tumours arising from connective tissues such as muscle, bone, cartilage and fat are termed sarcomas.

- Childhood tumours often occur if embryonic/foetal tissue is left behind. These tumours are named after the blastocyte from which cells and tissues are derived in the embryo, such as nephroblastoma and neuroblastoma.

- Sometimes the tissue of origin cannot be determined because the cells are undifferentiated tumours. These tumours are classified as primary of unknown origin.

Table 7: Tumour terminology related to tissue of origin

Tissue	Benign	Malignant
Epithelium	Papilloma	Carcinoma: basal cell carcinoma, squamous cell carcinoma, transitional cell carcinoma
Secretory or glandular epithelium	Adenoma	Adenocarcinoma
Connective		Sarcoma
Bone	Osteoma	Osteosarcoma
Cartilage	Chondroma	Chondrosarcoma
Fat	Lipoma	Liposarcoma
Fibrous	Fibroma	Fibrosarcoma
Voluntary muscles	Rhabdomyoma	Rhabdomyosarcoma
Involuntary muscles	Leiomyoma	Leiomyosarcoma
Tissue from foetal life		Blastoma

Locational

Often a type of cancer will be categorised by its location, for example cancer of the breast and cancer of the prostate. The actual site of any tumour is important in terms of symptoms, possible spread, treatment options and even prognosis. Treatment options will be different for a malignant melanoma of the retina compared with a malignant melanoma of the forearm. And a small tumour in the peripheral part of the lung may be treated differently to a tumour in the main bronchus.

Biological

Such a classification includes descriptions of the behaviour of the tumour, such as:

- Degree of differentiation (well, moderately, poorly, anaplastic)

  - As described earlier, the degree of differentiation (the grade) of a tumour is closely related to the potential metastasis. The more poorly differentiated the tumour is described as being, the greater the likelihood of metastasis. This is information that needs to be known at the outset of any patient management as it will help determine the most effective course of action.

- Lymphocyte positivity

  - Lymphocytes are a type of white blood cell that become active in response to a pathogen. They are an important part of the body's immune response. Tumours with infiltrating lymphocytes are recognised by the body, which then sets up an immune response. This lymphocyte positivity is often associated with increased response rates and better prognosis for cancer patients. Indeed, tumour-invading lymphocytes are being harvested and researched to form the basis of a newer, immunotherapeutic approach to cancer treatment.

- Hormone receptor status

  - Some tumours actively need hormones to survive. A woman's breast cancer might be referred to as oestrogen positive, ER+ve. Drugs such as tamoxifen and anastrozole (Arimidex®) are designed to inhibit the uptake of oestrogen by the breast cancer cell, either by blocking the receptor, in the case of tamoxifen, or inhibiting the conversion of androgens by aromatase in post-menopausal women, as is the case with anastrozole. Both drugs are designed to interfere with the uptake of oestrogen by the cancer cell thereby inhibiting its growth potential.

- Oncogene status

  - As describe earlier, cells are constantly receiving feedback and messages from their external environment, which stimulates them to grow and divide. Such messaging systems are known to be defective (permanently active) in most cancer cells. Knowledge of which messaging system is involved, and identification of the oncogenes (receptors on the cell surface) within that process that are abnormal, is leading the development of targeted drugs that can block the action of these proteins. One oncogene of particular note is the epidermal growth factor receptor (EGFR). EGFR has shown to be mutated in 90% of squamous cell carcinomas of the head and neck and 80% of colorectal cancers; it is also commonly mutated in many lung cancers. Such knowledge is helping to personalise care for those with cancer that express such mutations.

Tumour grade

The classifications described above create an assessment of the tumour, which affects the management options and prognosis of the patient. Tumours can also be categorised according to their grade and stage. Because all tumours are derived from a single rogue cell, it may be assumed that all subsequent cells should be identical or monoclonal; however, as the tumour cells continue to go through further cell cycles, they continue mutating so that a range of differentiations may be present within a tumour. The proportion of undifferentiated cells defines the grade of the tumour and provides an estimate on the degree of malignancy.

Generally, the grade is described on a scale of 1–4, as in table 8. Sometimes a tumour can be so markedly undifferentiated that it is difficult to ascertain the tissue of origin. These are referred to as anaplastic tumours and are generally highly malignant, offering the worst prognosis.

Table 8: The relationship between tumour grade and prognosis

Grade	Description	Prognosis
1	<25% undifferentiated cells	Better
2	>25%, <50% undifferentiated	↓
3	>50%, <75% undifferentiated	↓
4	>75% undifferentiated	Worse

For some tumour sites, it is necessary that a more accurate depiction of grade is assessed. An accurate assessment of grade in prostate cancer is essential in determining the treatment and possible outcome for men with this disease.

The grade for prostate cancer is obtained using the Gleason grading system. Multiple biopsies of the prostate are taken and the pathologist will look across the samples and assign scores based on the level of differentiation seen. Figure 16 shows a representation of differentiation patterns as described by Dr Gleason.

To assign the Gleason score, the pathologist will look across the samples and select a score to the most common pattern seen, for example pattern 3. The pathologist will then assign a score to the second most common pattern, for example 4. The 3 and 4 will be added together to give a total Gleason score of 7. This is often written 7 (3+4). Table 9 shows how the total Gleason score can be used to indicate the likely prognosis for patients with prostate cancer. A low Gleason score of 2–5 is usually defined as hyperplasia rather than cancer, and such low scores would probably indicate a watch and wait policy for treatment. Scores above 7 would indicate a malignant and potentially invasive disease that would require some form of intervention.

Figure 16: Diagrammatic representation of the Gleason grading system

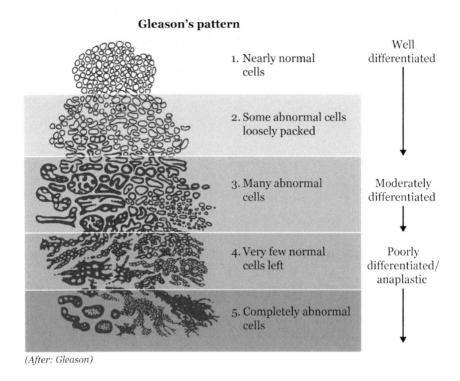

Gleason's pattern

1. Nearly normal cells — Well differentiated

2. Some abnormal cells loosely packed

3. Many abnormal cells — Moderately differentiated

4. Very few normal cells left — Poorly differentiated/ anaplastic

5. Completely abnormal cells

(After: Gleason)

Table 9: Interpretation of Gleason score

Gleason Score	Differentiation	Outlook and prognosis
2–5	Benign	Typical watch and wait policy
6	Well	Low grade; tends to grow and spread slowly; typical active surveillance policy
7	Moderate	
8–10	Poor	Aggressive disease; grows and spreads quickly

The tumour-node-metastasis (TNM) staging system developed jointly by the Union for International Cancer Control and the American Joint Committee on Cancer is widely recognised around the world as the principal staging system for most types of cancer. TNM forms the basis for cancer data collection within the UK as part of the National Cancer Data Repository and within US treatment facilities under the standards of the Commission on Cancer of the American College of Surgeons. Historically, there were many ways of staging different tumours, mainly dependent on the site within the body, which may lead to some confusion. Table 10 lists some of the other staging systems that are still used for certain primary cancers.

Table 10: Staging systems other than the TNM

Name of staging classification system	Tumours
Ann Arbor	Lymphomas (Hodgkin and non-Hodgkin)
The International Federation of Gynaecology and Obstetrics (FIGO)	Female gynaecological cancers: ovary, vagina and endometrial cervix
Dukes	Colorectal cancers

TNM staging describes the anatomic extent of the tumour; that is, how localised or how far spread the tumour is. It does this based on the assessment of three components:

- T – Extent of primary tumour

- N – Absence or presence and extent of regional lymph node involvement by the tumour

- M – Absence or presence of tumour at a distance from the primary site

By assigning numbers to these components (typically 0–4), an indication of the extent or severity of the disease can be made.

The T component represents the primary tumour and its size or extent at the site of origin. It can be classified according to the following general criteria:

- TX – Minimum requirements to assess the primary tumour cannot be met

- T0 – No evidence of primary tumour

- Tis – Carcinoma *in situ*

- T1–T4 – Progressive increase in tumour size and/or involvement of other structures

The definition of the T classification is relevant only for a particular tumour site and will vary. However, there are only two main ways in which tumour extension can be described: depth of invasion and size of tumour.

Depth of invasion tends to be used when the tumour site is located in a 'hollow' organ (see figure 17a), such as in the bladder, oesophagus or colon, where the organ typically has a lumen surrounded by layers of tissue, for example mucosa, submucosa, muscularis and serosa.

The size of the tumour tends to be used when the tumour site is located in a parenchymal (solid) organ (see figure 17b). Parenchymal organs, such as the liver, breast and lungs, have a specific function. Here, tumours will be described as being 2cm in the greatest diameter, for example.

Figure 17: T stage

(a) Hollow organs – e.g. bladder and colon

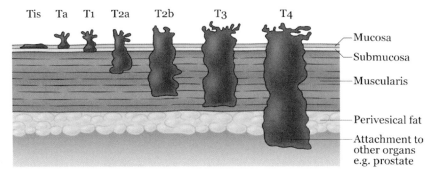

(b) Parenchymal (solid) organs – e.g. lungs, breast and liver

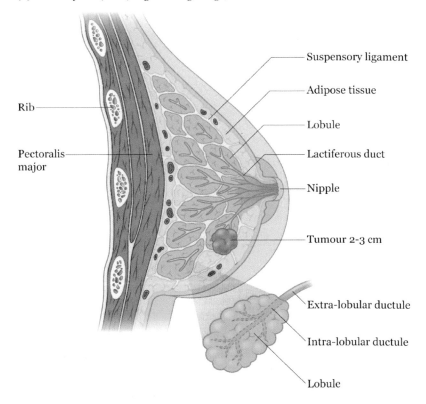

The N component describes regional lymph node involvement and can be categorised according to the following:

- Nx – Minimum requirements to assess the regional lymph nodes cannot be met

- N0 – No evidence of regional lymph node involvement

- N1–N3 – Increasing involvement of regional lymph nodes in size, number, location or other factors

It is important to note that the N category only applies to regional lymph nodes that are specifically listed in the TNM staging manual. Involvement of other distant nodes is classified in the M category.

The M category also describes the spread of the tumour via the blood to distant sites of the body.

- M0   – No evidence of distant metastases

- M1 – Presence of distant metastases

Additional notations may be added to highlight the site of the metastases, such as pulmonary (PUL), liver (HEP) and brain (BRA).

Each of these categories can be further annotated with a lowercase 'c' or 'p'. These refer to a clinical (c) stage and a pathological or post-surgical (p) stage.

Clinical stage (c)

A clinical stage is given based on evidence that can be seen through initial investigations. For example, a clinician may find a 2cm large tumour on a computerised tomography (CT) scan of a patient with a suspected lung cancer. The same scan may also reveal evidence of enlarged lymph nodes. Based on these clinical findings, this case can be given a clinical (c) stage.

The clinical stage suggests that lung cancer is present and surgery is needed to remove the tumour. The resection would then be sent to the pathology laboratory for further investigation by the pathologist.

Pathological (post-surgical) stage (p)

Further investigation by the pathologist might reveal that the tumour is in fact 5cm large and more lymph nodes are involved than was originally indicated. From this further analysis, the case is upstaged and the notation 'p' is used to describe this. The p stage indicates that further (adjunct) treatment is required.

Note here that, in case notes, the p is always present next to a pathological stage, for example pT1, whereas when stating the clinical stage, the c is mostly absent, for example T1.

Cancer registries throughout the world may also be aware of a third stage called the integrated stage, where a combination of the clinical and pathological stages is used to best represent the overall stage for this case.

Once the T, N and M categories have been noted, they are grouped together to give a stage. Excluding the X category, there are 48 different permutations of these components: T (0–4, is), N (0–3) and M (0–1). These permutations are assigned to broader categories called stage groups to give an indication of the likely prognosis and treatment strategy. Table 11 shows the stage grouping definitions for TNM.

Table 11: Stage group definitions

Stage classification	Stage group
Carcinoma in situ	0
Tumours localised to organ of origin	I & II
Locally extensive spread, particularly to local lymph nodes	III
Distant metastasis	IV

The classification of cancer, along with the stage and grade, forms the basis of an overall treatment plan for a specific case, which may comprise a combination of methods. The three main treatment strategies for cancer are surgery, radiotherapy and chemotherapy. Other therapies such as immunotherapy, hormone therapy and biological therapies also play an important role. In the following chapter, these different types of cancer treatment will be explored in further detail.

Chapter 4: Treatment of cancer

To be effective against cancer, a treatment plan must take into consideration the stage and grade of the disease. If detected at an early stage, the disease may be dealt with using a local treatment such as surgery. Whereas if it isn't identified until at a later stage, when the disease has metastasised, a more systemic approach to treatment such as chemotherapy is required. Likewise, patients deemed to have high grade tumours may be offered chemotherapy as the chance of metastasis is high. Whereas patients with low grade tumours have a low risk of metastasis, and therefore would need only a localised treatment. Below is a summary of the roles of each modality.

Surgery

Surgery plays an important role in both the treatment of cancer and in diagnosis and staging. It is a local treatment designed to remove all or part of the tumour at the primary site. Diagnostic samples (biopsies) can be removed and sent for further analysis to allow a histopathological diagnosis to be made. At the time of surgery, a sample may also be taken from the lymph nodes to see if they have any involvement, thereby providing information for the N classification. The extent of the primary tumour within the organ or tissue (T) can similarly be established.

Surgery as a treatment modality is able to control the primary tumour. It is also essential to recognise that many cancers may recur at the site of origin, making wide excision crucial in some cases. Recognition of the role of other therapies such as radiotherapy has, however, led to a more conservative approach to some surgical techniques. For example, in the early to mid-1900s, breast cancer was traditionally treated using a radical or total mastectomy. Clinical trials in the 1970s and 1980s demonstrated that this may not always be necessary and that local excision of the tumour followed by radiotherapy to the breast could offer as good a chance of cure while keeping the breast intact.

Radiotherapy

Radiotherapy is the treatment of cancer using high-energy ionising radiation. Ionising radiation is harmful to living tissue and, as such, it is necessary to control exposure to it. Again, it is predominantly a localised treatment, which can be broadly divided into two groups: external beam radiotherapy and brachytherapy.

External beam radiotherapy uses radiation that is created electronically by a linear accelerator, often referred to as a LINAC. Directed from a source outside the patient, the radiation aims to traverse the patient and deposit its energy in the tissue and tumour.

The deposition of energy inside the cell leads to the formation of free radicals, which are highly reactive agents that cause damage within the cell. Such damage (single and double strand DNA breaks) subsequently causes the cell to die.

The killing of cells with radiation is largely non-discriminatory. The radiation kills healthy cells as well as tumour cells, so care must be taken to ensure that little damage is received from normal healthy tissue. Careful planning is required to direct the radiation to the 'tumour volume', while at the same time making sure that the radiation dose is minimised so that it does not affect potential 'organs at risk'.

It is known that normal, otherwise healthy cells repair and recover from radiation damage more effectively than an abnormal, mutated tumour cell. This is the main reason why radiotherapy tends to be given in 'fractions' (a daily dose) over many days.

Figure 18 demonstrates how this works. Starting with 100% of cells (both healthy and tumourous) the first fraction (dose of radiation) is delivered. As radiation kills cells it can be expected that the lines will fall as cells die off. Notice how the normal cells die off at the same rate as the tumour cell – radiation will kill them both equally as well.

However, notice also that after waiting 24 hours the lines begin to rise. This is a result of normal and tumour cells recovering from the radiation damage. But the tumour line has not recovered quite as well as the normal cell line. When the next fraction is delivered, the lines drop again. The following process is repeated: fraction, drop, recover, fraction, drop, recover. And over the 25 or 30 fractions of radiotherapy, we will begin to see a difference in the rates of cell death. Figure 18 demonstrates how fractionation can be used to incrementally kill more tumour cells.

Figure 18: Fractionating radiotherapy

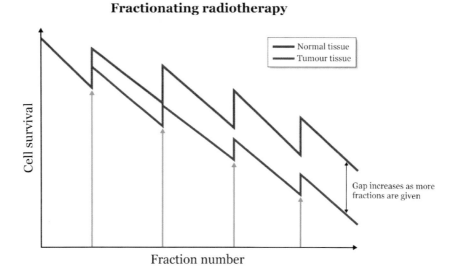

It is important to note that the normal cell line is dropping, just not quite as much. Thus, damage to normal tissue is still experienced and side effects will result. These include epilation (local hair loss), erythema (reddening of the skin like sunburn) and mucositis (inflammation of the mucous membrane, for example, in the mouth).

Brachytherapy (*brachys* = Greek for 'short range') is a medical treatment that involves the placement of small radioactive sources within a natural body cavity, through tissue or close to the surface. It is unlike the linear accelerator, where the radiation source disappears as soon as the device is switched off. Indeed, the physics behind brachytherapy means that the radiation is deposited in a short range of tissue, allowing high doses to be given to the tumour without necessarily irradiating too much healthy tissue. Brachytherapy can be administered in a variety of ways:

- Intracavity – the radioactive sources are placed into a cavity within the body, for example the uterus

- Intraluminal – the radioactive sources are placed into a lumen of the body, for example the oesophagus

- Interstitial – the radioactive sources are placed through tissue, for example implants for prostate cancer

Chemotherapy

Chemotherapy refers to the use of drugs to combat the disease process. More accurately, it should be referred to as cytotoxic chemotherapy because the drugs used to fight the cancer have a cytotoxic (cell killing) effect. Chemotherapy drugs work by halting or disrupting the normal cell cycle (see figure 2)

Different categories of chemotherapy drugs work in different ways, but they essentially stop DNA from forming or somehow interact directly with it, creating cross linkages and breaks. Either way, the cell fails to replicate and therefore dies.

Anti-metabolites

This category of drugs relies on the fact that the cell needs certain components to be able to function and replicate DNA. These can be divided into: purine (adenine and guanine) analogues; pyrimidine (thymine – or Uracil in RNA) and cytosine analogues; and antifolates.

Purines and pyrimidines are the essential building blocks of DNA, referred to as 'bases'. DNA is made up of a complex series of these bases, which are ordered in a certain way. A segment of the DNA containing these provides the instructions for producing proteins within the cell. Without the four bases – adenine, thymine, cytosine and guanine – DNA cannot replicate properly and the cell will die. Anti-metabolite chemotherapy drugs prevent these substances from being incorporated into the DNA, thereby stopping cell replication.

Antifolates are another group of drugs within this category. Folinic acid is required by the cell to allow the production of purines and pyrimidines. As seen above, these are the essential components of DNA. Antifolates work by impairing the function and production of folinic acid, thereby halting the production of purines and pyrimidines, which in turn stops cell replication and leads to cell death. Methotrexate is one example of an anti-metabolite chemotherapy drug that is used for a wide range of conditions, including psoriasis and rheumatoid arthritis. See table 12 for further examples of drugs within this category.

Table 12: Examples of anti-metabolite chemotherapy drugs

Purine analogues	Pyrimidine analogues	Antifolates
Mercaptopurine Thioguanine (used to treat acute leukaemias) Fludarabine Pentostatin and cladribine (adenosine analogues that are used primarily to treat hairy cell leukaemia)	5-fluorouracil (5FU) (inhibits thymidylate synthase)Cytosine arabinoside (Cytarabine, Ara-C) Gemcitabine	Methotrexate Pemetrexed

Alkylating agents

The nitrogenous bases of DNA join in a particular way. Adenine will only join onto thymine, while guanine will only join onto cytosine. Alkylating agent chemotherapy works by directly targeting DNA and causing bonds across bases where there should not be one. In particular, they are designed to produce covalent bonds between guanine bases. Such bonds interfere with DNA replication causing the cell to die.

Because this form of chemotherapy directly targets DNA, it is possible that the damaged cell tries to repair itself, or still replicates but in a damaged format. This is not ideal and may even lead to cancer, as alkylating agents are known carcinogens. Those who work in the coding world may be aware of the code (9920/3) in the International Classification of Diseases for Oncology (ICD-O3) diagnostics tool for therapy-related acute myeloid leukaemia, which includes a sub-bullet point for alkylating agent chemotherapy. It is possible for people to return with a second form of cancer possibly caused by the drugs given to them to cure them of an initial cancer.

Platinum-based drugs such as carboplatin and others are considered alkylating-like as they also cause bonds. However instead of using an 'alkyl' group they use a molecule of platinum to cause the bond between the guanine bases. The net result is the same, the cell struggles to replicate properly and dies. Examples of alkylating agent chemotherapy drugs can be seen in table 13.

Table 13: Alkylating agent chemotherapy (not exhaustive)

Alkylating agent	Alkylating-like
Cyclophosphamide	Cisplatin, Carboplatin, Oxaliplatin
Mechlorethamine or mustine (HN2) (trade name Mustardgen)Uramustine or uracil mustard	Satraplatin
Melphalan	
Chlorambucil	
Ifosfamide	
Carmustine	
Lomustine	
Streptozocin	
Busulfan	

Topoisomerase inhibitors

DNA is immensely long and needs to be tightly coiled and wound up to fit into the tiny nucleus. Therefore for the DNA to be able to replicate it needs to uncoil. An enzyme called topoisomerase (pronounced topo- isom- erase) allows this to happen. Indeed, without this enzyme to help uncoil DNA in an orderly fashion the DNA cannot splice apart easily and the cell will die.

There are two types of topoisomerase inhibitors, and these are designed to stop the DNA unwinding: topoisomerase I (topotecan, irinotecan) and topoisomerase II (etoposide, teniposide) inhibitors. Topoisomerase II inhibitors are also known carcinogens and, in a small number of cases, have put patients at risk of acquiring acute myeloid leukaemia two to three years after initial treatment.

Anti-tumour antibiotics

Common among these types of agents is their interference with cell division. Some are derived from bacteria and produce powerful free radicals, which damage the DNA of the cell and cause cell death.

The anthracyclines are a particularly notable class of anti-tumour antibiotics, which include drugs such as doxorubicin (Adriamycin), idarubicin and epirubicin. Such drugs are known to cause damage to the heart and often come with a lifetime dose limit. Patients receiving these drugs are assessed and monitored for heart problems before and after receiving treatment. Other (non-anthracycline) drugs in this category would include bleomycin, mitomycin and actinomycin.

Mitotic inhibitors

When a cell is ready to divide, it enters the mitosis phase of the cell cycle. As the cell begins to cleave apart, the two new cells are momentarily joined by the formation of microtubules. Once the cell is completely satisfied that division can occur, the microtubules are disassembled and two separated cells result.

Two groups of mitotic inhibitor drugs prevent this cell division from occurring: vinca alkaloids and taxanes. But their mechanisms of action are juxtaposed.

Vinca alkaloids

Originally harvested and derived from the Periwinkle plant, vinca alkaloids bind to tubulin and interfere with the assembly of the microtubules. The original vinca alkaloids include vincristine and vinblastine. Other semi-synthetic drugs now exist such as vinorelbine, vindesine and vinflunine.

Taxanes

These drugs were also harvested from natural sources, for example the first, paclitaxel, was derived from the Pacific Yew Tree. Now, paclitaxel (as well as another taxane called docetaxel) is produced semi-synthetically. In contrast to vinca alkaloids, these drugs promote microtubule stability, which prevents their disassembly. The net result is the same, the cell cannot cleave apart and will therefore die.

Like radiotherapy, chemotherapy is given in discrete bouts of treatment, referred to as cycles. A full cycle of chemotherapy comprises the time taken to give the drugs along with a rest period for the patient. Within a typical cycle length of 21 days, the drugs tend to be administered between days one and five (D1-5). The patient will then have 16 days' rest before receiving the next dose of chemotherapy. The second cycle starts again at D1.

Cycles of chemotherapy work on the same basis as radiotherapy fractionation. The rest period allows the human body to recover just enough to tolerate the next dose of chemotherapy. Although this time also allows tumour tissue to recover, as mentioned previously, normal cells recover better than tumour cells. Once again, this differential can be accentuated over a number of cycles.

Also like radiotherapy, chemotherapy drugs are non-discriminatory; they affect healthy cells as well as tumour cells and therefore side effects can occur (see table 14). Generally, the more frequently a cell divides, the more sensitive it is to the chemotherapy drug, which is why noted side effects tend to occur in those areas of the body with fast-dividing tissue, such as in mucous membranes, the digestive tract and bone marrow.

Biological (targeted) therapy

Radiotherapy and chemotherapy are powerful treatment strategies designed to kill tumour cells effectively. However, they also do too much damage to the healthy tissue and patient, which is why many people, for example lymphoedema nurses, are employed in hospitals and clinics to deal with the after effects of treatment rather than the cancer itself.

Table 14: Common side effects of chemotherapy

General	Organ specific
Bone marrow suppression Hair loss – alopecia Nausea and vomiting Appetite and weight loss Taste changes Sores in mouth and throat Fatigue	Heart damage (cardiac toxicity) – daunorubicin and doxorubicin Nervous system changes – mitotic inhibitors, vincristine Lung damage (pneumotoxicity) – bleomycin Liver and kidney damage Secondary cancers

This is partly because radiotherapy and chemotherapy do not really pay attention to the differences between healthy cells and tumours cells. A difference is manufactured in radiotherapy through using different angled beams, conformal and intensity modulated radiotherapy, as well as fractionation. With regards to chemotherapy, cancer patients sometimes receive a combination of drugs that have different modes of action and side effects. By using these strategies, an incrementally greater effect of radiotherapy and chemotherapy on tumours over healthy cells can be manufactured.

Contrastingly, biological therapies consider the difference between tumour cells and normal cells. As described in chapter one, all cells rely on a signalling pathway that converts messages (which usually come from outside the cell) to actions: the cell will grow, it will divide, it may move and it may die. In cancer, this signalling pathway is disrupted by damage and mutation, which can lead to aberrant and incorrect messages being received. Herein lie the differences between tumour cells and normal cells... but what exactly are their distinguishing characteristics?

Figure 19 demonstrates how a cancer cell can be differentiated from a normal cell, and table 15 shows how these differences can be further divided into targets that appear on the outside of the cell (extracellular) and those that appear on the inside of the cell (intracellular).

Figure 19: What makes a cancer cell different?

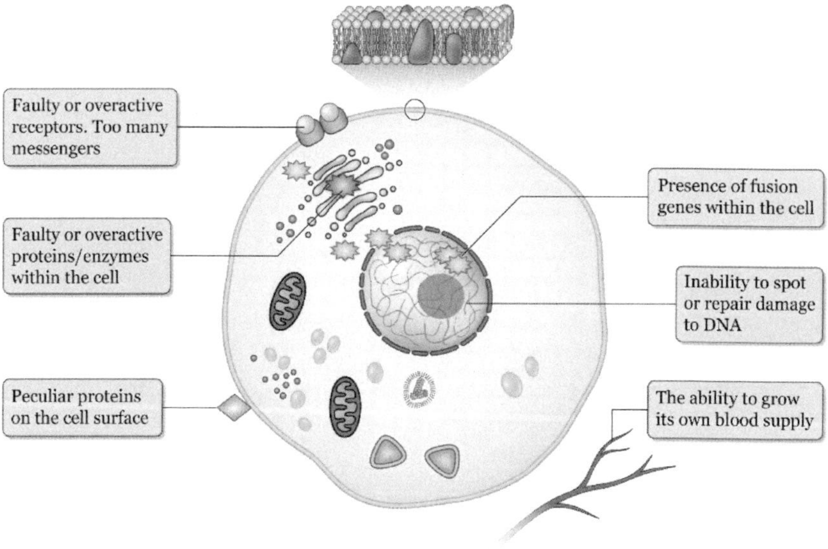

Faulty or overactive receptors. Too many messengers

Faulty or overactive proteins/enzymes within the cell

Peculiar proteins on the cell surface

Presence of fusion genes within the cell

Inability to spot or repair damage to DNA

The ability to grow its own blood supply

Table 15: Extracellular and intracellular differences of a cancer cell

Extracellular differences / targets	Intracellular differences / targets
• Too many ligands (messengers) – epidermal growth factor; vascular epithelial growth factor • Overactive receptor – epidermal growth factor receptor • Overexpression of receptor – HER2 (breast cancer) • Peculiar proteins on cell surface – CD20, CD30, CD52	• Mutation in a signalling protein so that it is constitutively active – keeps telling cell to divide even in the absence of the message (BRAF, KRAS) • Mutation in the DNA machinery –fusion genes (Philadelphia chromosome in chronic myeloid leukaemia; Anaplastic lymphoma kinase (ALK) in lung cancer) • Tumour suppressor genes not working (p53, PTEN, Rb)

Extracellular targets

Too many ligands (messengers)

All cells rely on messages being received and interpreted. Cancer cells produce many messages (growth factors), which influence other cancer cells around them to grow and proliferate. As described earlier, a tumour only has to grow a few millimetres in diameter before it needs more oxygen, which it will derive from creating a new blood supply (angiogenesis).

A powerful stimulant of angiogenesis is vascular endothelial growth factor (VEGF). Tumour cells will secrete vast quantities of VEGF, which will interact with nearby blood vessels, promoting growth of new blood vessels that will feed the tumour.

New angiogenesis inhibitor drugs, such as bevacizumab (Avastin) and sorafenib inhibit the attachment of VEGF onto the endothelial (cells lining the blood vessel walls), thereby stopping the message to produce a new blood vessel.

Such an approach is designed to prevent blood vessel formation in and around the tumour, starving it of oxygen and nutrients, and limiting a potential route for metastasis. Unfortunately, blood vessel formation is also important in many normal body processes, such as wound healing, heart and kidney function, foetal development and reproduction. Side effects of treatment with angiogenesis inhibitors can include problems with bleeding, clots in the arteries (with resultant stroke or heart attack), hypertension and protein in the urine.

Overactive receptor and overexpression of receptor

In some cancers, a cell surface receptor can be overactive, meaning it is permanently in the 'on' state and transmitting messages to the cell even in the absence of a growth factor. The epidermal growth factor receptor (EGFR) is known to be overactive in many colorectal cancers and squamous cell carcinomas of the head and neck. Drugs such as cetuximab (Erbitux) and panitumumab (Vectibix) attach to the extracellular portion of EGFR and block the binding site for the growth factor (message). Small molecule inhibitors, such as gefitinib, erlotinib, brigatinib and lapatinib, bind to the intracellular portion of EGFR. Such binding prevents EGFR from activation, which is a prerequisite for the binding of downstream adaptor proteins. This results in the halting of the signalling cascade in cells that rely on the pathway for growth, tumour proliferation and migration.

HER2 (neu, ERB2) is an example of a receptor that is often over expressed on the surface of breast cancer cells. Damage to the genes of the cell may mean that when the cell replicated it produced too many HER2 receptors. As a result, the cell will naturally receive too many messages to divide, proliferate and potentially metastasise. Trastuzumab (Herceptin) attaches to HER2 and blocks its action. Pertuzumab (Perjeta) can also block its action, but in a slightly different way, by preventing the dimerization (coming together) of the two receptors.

Peculiar proteins on the cell surface

Some cancers will express a particular protein on the surface of the cell that can be used as a target. For example, most follicular non-Hodgkin lymphomas will express CD20, which is the target for rituximab (Rituxan, MabThera). Rituximab works by attracting and improving the work of T cells in destroying these cells. Ofatumumab, ocrelizumab and obinutuzumab are examples of other drugs that target the CD20 proteins on cancer cells.

Intracellular targets

It is also possible to target the internal portion of an overactive receptor. small molecule inhibitors such as gefitinib are designed to target the internal portion of EGFR in lung cancers that are EGFR +ve (about 10–15%).

Mutation in a signalling protein

It is known that with some cancers there can be damage (a mutation) in the proteins that transfer messages to the nucleus. These signalling proteins, including BRAF, KRAS and MEK, are known to be mutated in certain cancers, such that the signalling pathway is constitutively active, even in the absence of a ligand / receptor interaction. Half of malignant melanomas have BRAF mutations, and drugs like vemurafenib and dabrafenib are designed to inhibit the action of this mutated protein.

Mutation in the DNA machinery

Such mutation can fall into two categories: the creation of fusion genes and the disruption of tumour suppressor genes such as P53, RB and PTEN.

Genetic events, including gene translocations and deletions, can cause the formation of fusion genes, whereby two previously separate genes are rearranged to create a hybrid gene. The Philadelphia chromosome is one example of such a gene, and while it is generally associated with chronic myeloid leukaemia, it can also be seen in other types of leukaemia and lymphoma. The Philadelphia chromosome, or BCR / ABL, is a fusion gene that results when a portion of chromosome 22 and a portion of chromosome 9 swap over (translocation) (see figure 20).

The Philadelphia chromosome promotes white blood cell growth and replication; it is the driving force behind chronic myeloid leukaemia. Drugs such as imatinib, dasatinib, nilotinib and, more recently, radotinib and bosutinib, are designed to combat the action of this fusion gene and halt the progress of the disease.

Tumour suppressor genes play an important role in preventing cancer from occurring in our cells. Such genes are responsible for monitoring whether damage occurs within the cell (DNA) and facilitating repair. If repair cannot be achieved, then the tumour suppressor gene may initiate apoptosis (programmed cell death). These types of genes protect the cell from progressing on the path towards cancer. Therefore, if they mutate, causing a loss or reduction in their function, the cell can then become cancerous. Other factors, as discussed earlier, are also required to enable cancer to fully develop, but tumour suppressor genes are crucial in this whole turn of events. Failure to develop treatment strategies to reinsert tumour suppressor genes, or to make them operative once again, means that targeting tumour suppressor genes with effective treatment has so far eluded scientists.

Figure 20: Philadelphia chromosome

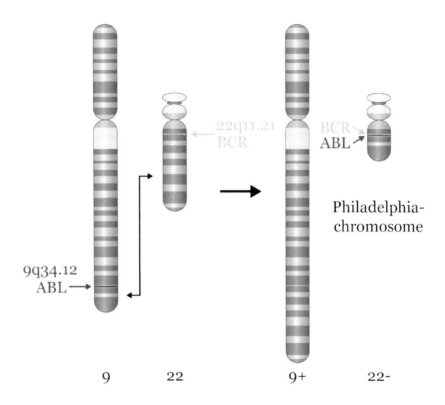

Biological (targeted) therapies use monoclonal antibodies (mAbs) and small molecule inhibitors to target the mutated protein. Monoclonal antibodies are large structures (comparatively) and any target needs to be extracellular (on a surface or ligand). It also needs to be big enough for the mAb to bind to (such as a protein) and something that the cell needs to survive. If the mAb is designed to attract immune cells, as is the case with rituximab, then there needs to be immune cells present in and around the tumour. Furthermore, any target needs to present, ideally, only on cancer cells, or at least be over expressed (have too many copies of the receptor) on the cancer cell.

Small molecule inhibitors, on the other hand, are small enough to enter through the cell membrane and interact (compete for) binding sites within the cell itself. As many of the binding sites within the signal cascade are similar, small molecule inhibitors tend to be less specific and can possibly interact with several targets.

The term 'targeted' therapy therefore becomes a bit of a misnomer and needs further clarification. The presence of receptors and the use of the signal cascade is a process that is normal and common to all cells within the body. The fact that they are mutated (over expressed) in cancer cells make them a useful target, but not an exclusive one. The net result is that patients still experience side effects.

Many targeted therapy drugs cause a rash or other skin changes that can range from mild to severe. Skin problems occur because many of the drugs used target aberrant EGFR, which is mutated in many cancers and is a useful target. But EGFR is found naturally on many other cells within the body. For example, epithelial cells of the skin have many EGF receptors and, as such, are quickly damaged by drugs (e.g. cetuximab and erlotinib) that target this receptor in EGFR +ve disease.

Interestingly, it has been demonstrated that certain side effects may be associated with a better patient outcome. For example, patients who develop acneiform rash (skin eruptions that resemble acne) while being treated with the inhibitors erlotinib or gefitinib have tended to respond better to these drugs than patients who do not develop the rash. Table 16 lists some common and less common side effects of targeted treatments.

Table 16: Side effects to targeted therapies

Side effects	Comments
Skin	More common with EGFR targeted therapy; can range from dry skin to severe acne, which is itchy and sore
High blood pressure	Anti-angiogenic drugs
Bleeding or blood clotting problems	Anti-angiogenic drugs can cause bruising and bleeding; internal bleeding can be life threatening
Slow wound healing	Anti-angiogenic drugs can interfere with wound healing, such as old wounds opening and new wounds not closing; can also lead to perforations in the stomach or intestine
Autoimmune reactions	Checkpoint inhibitors (more detail on these later) may take the brakes off the immune system, allowing it to attack the body's own cells and tissues
Other side effects	Nausea and vomiting; diarrhoea or constipation; mouth sores

Immunotherapy

Immunotherapy is the name given to treatments that initiate the body to fight against cancer. These types of drugs are sometimes referred to as biological response modifiers because they promote the body's own response to fight an infection (in this case cancer). Immunotherapy can be local – as in the treatment of carcinoma of the bladder, where Bacillus of Calmete and Guerin (BCG) is administered directly into the bladder via a catheter – or it can be systemic, where the drug is used to treat the whole body, such as interferon or interleukin 2, which have been shown to be effective against kidney cancer. Moreover, immunotherapy drugs can be given to boost the body's natural defence system (termed non-specific immunotherapy) or they can be used to target individual tumour cells. Such an approach tends to use monoclonal antibodies.

To appreciate how monoclonal antibodies can be used in an immunotherapy approach to cancer treatment, it is first necessary to look at how the immune system works in relation to cancer. At the beginning of this book the hallmarks of cancer were listed, including two further hallmarks that were added in 2011. One of these was the tumour's ability to evade the body's immune system. Immune cells (T cells) scan the body's other cells and tissues, searching for foreign bodies, bacteria, viruses and cancer cells. As the T cell approaches a normal body cell there is an interaction in which the normal cell is 'seen' as normal by the T cell and left alone. The T cell probes for certain proteins that serve as identifying markers for healthy, normal cells. If the proteins indicate that the cell is infected or cancerous, the T cell will lead an attack against it.

Programmed cell death 1 (PD-1) and cytotoxic T-lymphocyte associated protein 4 (CTLA-4) are the probes that the T-cell uses to seek out infected or cancerous cells. Programmed cell death ligand 1 (PD-L1) is the protein on the normal cell that interacts with PD-1 and indicates to the T cell to leave it alone. Such an interaction is called a checkpoint and is analogous to a 'molecular handshake', indicating that all is well.

However, it appears that cancer cells are also good at producing proteins such as PD-L1. The result being that when a circulating T cell comes across a cancerous cell, which expresses PD-L1, the molecular handshake takes place and fools the T cell into thinking the cancer cell is in fact a normal cell and can be left alone.

A range of drugs called checkpoint inhibitors can either block these normal proteins on cancer cells or the proteins on T cells that respond to them. Consequently, this removes the molecular handshake that prevents T cells from recognising the cells as cancerous and allows for an immune system assault on the cancer cells.

Three monoclonal antibodies, checkpoint inhibitors, have recently received approval for use: ipilimumab (PD-1), pembrolizumab (PD-1) and nivolumab (CTLA-4). These block the molecular handshake by interacting directly with the T cell probe. Atezolizumab is another checkpoint inhibitor, however this drug interacts with PD-L1 found on the antigen-presenting cell. Figure 21 shows the interaction of these drugs with T cells and cancer cells.

Figure 21: Checkpoint inhibitors

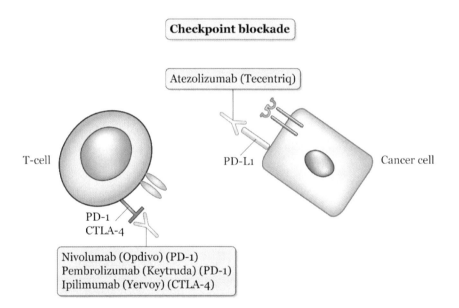

These and other immune checkpoint therapies represent one of the most promising of cancer treatment strategies to date, with encouraging results found in patients with advanced melanoma and lymphoma.

A word of caution, however. By releasing the brakes on the immune system, the molecular handshake for all cells can potentially be withdrawn. This is a crucial protective mechanism that stops T cells from attacking healthy, normal cells, and without it normal body cells are potentially open to attack from the immune system, which could cause catastrophic autoimmune-type responses. Common side effects include fatigue, cough, nausea, loss of appetite, skin rash and itching. More serious problems might be seen in the lungs, intestines, liver, kidneys, hormone-making glands and other organs.

The multidisciplinary approach to the treatment of cancer

Much has been done over the past decade to bring groups of professionals together to focus on improving treatment for individual cancer patients. These multidisciplinary teams comprise diverse disciplines that provide comprehensive assessment and consultation for a particular cancer case. While primarily there to help team members resolve difficult cases, teams may also fulfil a variety of additional functions. For example, they can help promote coordination between different professionals; provide a 'checks and balances' mechanism to ensure that the interests and rights of all concerned parties (particularly the patient) are addressed; and perhaps identify service gaps and breakdowns in coordination or communication. They also enhance the professional skills and knowledge of individual team members by providing a forum for learning more about different strategies, resources and approaches used across various disciplines for cancer treatment. Such an approach to the treatment of individual cancer cases is essential for providing appropriate management strategies and attaining the best possible chance of cure for the patient.

Conclusion

Huge strides have been made to improve cancer treatments in recent years, which has led to more people surviving cancer than ever before. In the UK today, over 85% of women survive breast cancer for five years or more, compared with just over 50% in the early 1970s. The commencement of the cervical screening programme in the UK and Europe has seen a dramatic decrease in the number of women presenting with invasive cancers of the cervix. And our development of excellent treatments for acute lymphoblastic leukaemia and nephroblastoma means that most children diagnosed with the disease are able to survive their battle.

Unfortunately, there are certain types of cancer, such as lung and pancreatic, where survival rates remain low, with the search for effective treatments proving more complicated and challenging. But even in these areas, improvements are slowly being made through ongoing research and education.

Treatment advances and prevention strategies are undoubtedly continuing to tackle the disease. However, the world's population is living for longer – with many in developing countries expected to live above 90 years of age – and this, combined with the fact that most people diagnosed with cancer are 60 years of age and above, is having an inevitable impact on cancer rates.

In 2015, the World Health Organization warned of a worldwide cancer epidemic, with numbers of cases expected to increase by around 50% in the next 20 years. Although the developing world will experience its share of the disease, developing countries within Africa, Asia and South America will begin to see an ever-increasing number of cancer cases, perhaps without the health services required to deal with such numbers.

It begs the question: can we cure our way out of this situation? If we use the knowledge gained about the hallmarks of cancer then maybe we can. But as highlighted in this book, cancer is not just one disease. It may well be that we have to find over 200 cures.

Perhaps a way can be found to reinsert tumour suppressor genes into tumour cells, thereby utilising a cell's natural defence mechanism against mutations. Work is already underway to harness one's own immune system to fight cancer. But while this has great potential, it also comes with great risk. Learning more about the immune system and how it can be used to fight cancer is essential for progress to be made in this area.

It may be that prevention is a more favourable way forward. Vaccination schemes for the human papillomavirus (HPV), for example, are proving extremely useful against cervical cancer. Such preventive strategies may be a promising route for other types of cancer too, and rolling these schemes out across developing countries will play a significant role in protecting against cancer worldwide.

Early diagnosis saves lives where cancer is concerned, therefore a huge emphasis is placed on making people aware of cancer and the risks associated with its development. Informing people about the signs and symptoms of cancer may prompt many to seek medical advice earlier than they do at present, leading to more cancers being diagnosed at an early stage when treatments are likely to be more successful. Many schemes have been introduced to raise awareness of key contributors such as unhealthy eating, smoking, alcohol and sun exposure. However, these initiatives will take time to bear fruit, and governments need to keep such educational activities at the forefront of the agenda for effective results to be seen in the future.

Reducing the risk of cancer when we are older starts with good habits when we are young. It is imperative that healthy lifestyle initiatives designed to highlight cancer risks include a specific focus on children and adolescents, ensuring that this demographic has a healthy respect for the disease without fearing it. Giving young people the information necessary to make educated, informed decisions about their risk of developing cancer is crucial. But how this information is communicated to young people in a way that is palatable and clear to them needs more research and enterprise than is currently available. If we can get our education strategy towards young people right, we will reduce cancer risk at an older age and hopefully put a brake on the ever-increasing incidence of cancer diagnoses.

About David O'Halloran

David provides cancer training and educational resources developed specifically for individuals and teams working within cancer related environments.

He is passionate about **empowering people through learning** and believes that insight and understanding is fundamental for people working in a cancer related field and we're passionate about cancer.

Originally trained as a therapeutic radiographer, he quickly became involved in teaching about cancer and was a senior lecturer in radiotherapy at the University of Leeds.

Since 2002 David has worked as a cancer education and training specialist delivering courses throughout the UK to various cancer organisations; NHS, Cancer Charities, Pharmaceutical companies and others.

David also delivers webinars, internet lecturers designed to bring high quality training and education without the need for travel.

Find out more about these courses and webinars at www.ohconsultancy.co.uk

Made in the USA
San Bernardino, CA
02 June 2020

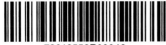